All 3 Resurgence in one collection.

Resurgence

From Stroke to Life.

Author: Peter. T. Raven.

This is based on real events.

First of all, let me tell you a little bit about

Myself and what this story is all about.

My name is Peter. and I am 46årOld at the time of writing.

This story is about what happened

in my life and how it affects my everyday life at present.

Okay Then We Begin!

I take you back to the 21 July 2012 which

was the day when everything changed.

I am the father of four sons, two of which are resident

in Karlstad.

Firstly, I would like to mention that when this

took place, I was homeless and lived in

My car for several months.

So, 21 July, a very hot and sunny day in

lovely Karlstad and I had
spent an entire

week with my beautiful sons

In this beautiful day, me and
my sons had

 gone inline skating around
the city and along the

the water where there are beautiful walkways to go on.

We had been and had coffee at a café in the city center

and the clock began approaching 17 o'clock in the afternoon, so we decided to go back

Then the boys would eat food at that time.

The return trip went without incident, but I

began to feel strangely tired.

The boys would go in and eat the food and I said

I go to the Cape and putting me to rests,

A few hours so we hear of later.

We parted at 17.30 hours and I was driving and

parked at the Cape, put me in the back seat and fell asleep.

When I woke up again had the dark

presented themselves and the time showed 22.45 hrs. and my son

Had sent a text message to me.

I tried to focus on what he wrote but

had a little hard to decipher what it was, but

managed to finally see that he wondered what I did.

I tried to talk to him and
managed to get

off two text messages before I
noticed that my right arm fell
to the floor of my car.

I was amazed and first
thought that struck

me was that my shoulder had
fallen asleep in the half

Prone position I was in.

I lifted up my right arm again and

Started a new text message to my son.

Suddenly thump and my right arm had once again landed on the floor of the car.

I thought it was strange
because I did not

To the fallen down on the
floor again.

In the same moment I stared
at my phone

and SMS I would send to my
son included

just a bunch of letters, no
coherent at all.

It struck me as odd because I know

I typed text.

I felt I had to try to sit

me up and would drive down the right leg against

the floor in order to be able to do it, but what? Me right leg did not budge either!

Now I started to understand what was

Happening and I knew my time was getting very limited.

With one last effort, I called up my son.

I tried to tell him that they have to

send an ambulance
immediately because I have a
stroke.

My son was scared and
confused and left

the phone to his foster father
and I tried

repeat that I got a stroke and
needed a

ambulance immediately.

My son's foster father said to me that they would

come and pick me up instead because it

would go faster than it would take for

The ambulance to reach me.

We put on and I knew they were going to

me.

In the meantime, I was waiting I thought much on

My life, it looked like images in my mind.

Damn this cannot happen to me I was thinking

at the same time that I was sorry and fought

In order not to burn out.

I thought the time was standing still, I felt dizzy

and faint, realized that I had to get up

and get out of the car to the fresh air,

While I was waiting for my son and his foster father.

"I was really worried about you when it came

thought you would die.

I been completely gone because I never have been through this before, but I cried much and I panicked.

This is my son's own statements and they speak for themselves.

With my last power I used left

arm and the left leg to sometimes lag,

Alternately pull myself out of the car and tried to best I could to set me upright against the car.

When I finally succeeded with
this huge

feat, to stand upright outside
the car and

wait for help, I felt a little
more alert, but

at the same time, I felt at that
time the facial paralysis

On the right side seriously.

I stood and wobbled a bit
back and forth

because of fatigue and
exhaustion, when I

Finally saw a car came driving
towards me.

Finally had my beloved son come to the rescue.

He came rushing towards me, scared and with the tears flowing.

He tried to help me, but due to

the right side of the body was completely paralyzed became

I simply too heavy for a 16-year-old.

So his foster father drove his car

further, then walked up to me and took a

hug-on me, and lifted me into the back seat of his,

car and the ride to the hospital began.

This trip I never forget.

The body wanted to stop
breathing and pictures out of
my life

passed in Revue and in the
distance I heard someone

scream that I have to stay
awake and I have to talk all
the time.

I could in my condition not
determine who was yelling or
why.

My only thought was that I must survive at any price.

When we finally arrived at the emergency intake on

Karlstad's hospital staff stood and waited for us.

I was immediately transferred to an emergency

stretcher and was rolled in for treatment.

During the first day I had time with two skull

x-ray and clot-busting agents introduced

Intravenously for an hour's time.

The first day was brought I was woke up every 15th minutes

For blood pressure and blood sugar shooting and each

time I got to speak with the staff so they saw that

I was contactable.

After this gruesome first day I felt

me as a total package because I had not

slept, several blood tests and

Medical examinations.

The only thing I could think of was my kids

And that I must live for their sake.

So I decided to fight.

On my 3rd day I had stabilized so that

they could move me by taxi to Karlskoga

Hospital and checking on Department 1A which

Is a pure stroke ward.

There it became more skull x-ray.

I had to spend the first night in

monitoring and blood pressure shooting day two,

revealed staff to the two scull x-ray

from Karlstad not shown any results and not the one made in Karlskoga.

This puzzled the doctors and the

decided that a magnet x-ray was only

option that could reveal where this

cerebral infarction started.

Said and done, in the evening,
I was brought

to magnetic camera which is
like a big

Tin drum which you go into
on a bunk.

This monster will check
through your brain with

a variety of methods including

High frequency sounds.

After such an inquiry, it feels like

the brain was left in the machine sounds

Spinning around in my head the rest of the day.

On rounds day after the doctor wanted to speak with me.

He explained that they found the plug/

attack and according to the doctor he could see on,

The pictures that I was big smoker ha-ha.

Why I find it funny?

Well because I never smoked more than five cigarettes per day ever.

But after reading a lot about stroke on the internet

 so I too realized that smoking is actually a killing factor.

So I decided to quit smoking.

I can't cross stop but I can stair

Down to 4 a day to begin with.

After these tours with various tests

I thought I finally come to the stage

I would take it easy and
collect me.

It turned out to be completely
wrong!

Now it was time for a new
poll and

This time it was about test

Of the neck by means of x-
rays.

Back to the couch and then
lying completely still

so the nurse slowly and carefully, could

examine every millimeter of the neck muscles

and blood circulation.

This study is to see if.

There is constriction of the blood vessels or on the breathing.

There is a risk that muscles become swollen and causes

Problems with food or
breathing.

It turned out to be all right.

"Nice" so now at last I get to

Room and rest, I thought.

But now had second thoughts
about health care

the situation.

Now it was time for sick gymnasts to come

into the picture!

These people present themselves in a very

friendly and nice way and declare that they

Will help me to get started with my training.

I should add that I myself worked in the medic line of work when Younger.

medic care and in particular with orthopedics and

Psychiatry.

So my gymnasts asked me to go with them

down to the gymnastics to try out a

wheelchair and a crutch that will be

My companion on the road.

We started my work out that included that

get up on the legs and
touching on both the legs.

Also included is facial
gymnastics in scheduling.

For the first time since the
stroke, I should now

try to stand on both legs,
which is a terrible effort.

Trying to drive me in to the
rail system which is a steel

construction with two rails
and plates

Hold them together at the
bottom.

I try to stand still but the body
would fall to the right!

 I try to concentrate, try to get

balance in the body and
manages to stand still

without knowing that I would
fall what happiness!

My sick gymnasts watching
me, smiling and

Call on me to take a step forward.

I stare at them and they nod and say "

Come on you can do it".

I grip the left railing hard and staring

down on my right foot and try to get it to take a step forward.

Watching and sends the signal to the foot and leg but nothing happens!

The staff told me to start with the left

feet, which would mean that I
am forced

Stressing the right leg to be
able to move forward the left.

Jeez, man becomes fearful
and hesitant but I

Tell me that I can do it.

With determined my starts I move the weight

to the right leg and know the importance of the hip

And thighs on the right side, but dare I?

I move quickly forward with left foot, regain

balance and feel really proud.

I managed to distribute the weight, the staff will be

And waiting and I ask what they are waiting for?

They respond and now do the same thing with right leg!

But how then? I thought to myself

But staring down on the leg
and foot and

really tried to force a motion
of any kind.

I stood for a long time, a very
long time and tried to

forcing my foot or leg to move
forward

but nothing happened!

But all of a sudden!

Oh the leg moves forward, actually very slow

And trailing but it is actually moving forward!

What a great feeling.

I get the legs next to each other again and

the staff says "very good job" and I feel so proud.

The staff tells me to put me in

The wheelchair again because it may be enough for today.

I get help from staff to the Division.

We end with evening snacks or make up to

every day Monday through
Friday should I work out two

hours to get as much
movement in

My arm and my leg as
possible.

The following days along the
same pattern and

the leg begins to move more
every day

and things are going better
and better to go forward

With the help of the needles.

When will the next mortal blow from the staff.

Today P, try to go with the help of a crutch!

I thought ' help, how the hell should I succeed with

This? ", but at the same time, I saw it as a challenge.

Of course I have to learn to walk with a crutch!

I got a crutch as they
adjusted to the right length

and was told to go on me,
which I did.

I was fading a bit before I got

body in balance.

I tentatively moved up the left
foot and

Then I tried to follow suit with
the right leg.

Then suddenly it happened
that did not happen, I got

fell head over heels to the right and landed in a pile on

the floor.

The staff rushed out to check on if I injured myself.

They wanted to help me up but I shouted ' no '.

I said I can get up myself and did everything

I could come up with to take me up again,

But I managed to not, unfortunately.

So the staff helped me up in the wheelchair again

, which is defeat!

This made me downright pissed.

My body is so strong, not
even go

forward with a crutch!

The staff was trying to tell me
to calm but I

replied only that I want them
to help me

to practice to get up from
lying down

Position on the floor itself.

If it happens once, it can happen more was my train of thought.

They promised to begin the exercise the same

Afternoon and so was the case.

Lying on the floor, on the right side, not

Neither the movement nor sensation.

Do like this: with the left arm push yourself up in

Sitting position, try to get balance.

When you can sit without falling back, fold

right leg toward the left so you get into

tailors position, then try to fold

the left leg so that you can get up on left knee.

 With the left knee to the floor to take the support of the left

arm and try also to get up on it

right knee "absolutely not easy I know".

Now with the help of the left leg and left arm

push yourself up to a Chair or wheelchair, and you

have now managed to get up off the floor at your own care.

After this day, I was firmly determined I

To go and I won't fall any
more time!

The following days I struggled
as a possessed and

managed to get the legs and
feet more and more but

noticed another strange thing
with

Right foot.

I knew neither the toes or heel and foot wanted

Does not come with wiggle position in points either.

Very odd.

Spoke with the staff about this phenomenon and the

would send referral to orthopedic technician

a foot frame that helps direct the foot

Forward and also keeps it firmly against the floor.

 Said and done, an appointment with the technician showed up

a few days later and I got to try out and

Jeez what a difference!

Staff had also ordered a brand new

Wheel chair for me which was my own and even a

brand new crutch.

Now started training seriously.

But a concern remained.

The arm, what about your arm?

Could say as much to the arm has been trained in

the extent of the leg and the foot but

Unfortunately, without any results.

There is very little sensation
in fingertips but that's all.

No movement at all but it
hangs more or

less there as ornament.

 So my priority is that you will
understand right

leg and foot.

Meanwhile, the Department
1a, I have trained

incessantly and had decent time both with

crutch and behold, even shorter distances without!

In section 1A in Karlskoga, I was under the

more than 2.5 weeks, my days consisted of training

and outdoor training for exercise and strength

Every day the whole weeks.

I was released from the ward 1A

 8 August and I was moved to a short-term

accommodation in Degerfors
municipality, which is

The end of the world really.

Wherever you are it is uphill
slopes and

sitting in a wheelchair, there
is no further arrangement

with slopes everywhere.

My training has continued and consists at present

of both the arm, hand, leg.

I go every day so much I just can't be bothered

To be able to get to as good time as possible.

Physical training of arm and joints is to

Maintain the softness and bending ability of all joints.

Today, on August 22 and it will soon be

past five weeks ago since the stroke and I

feel refreshed and alert and ready for new

challenges.

This is the story to date, but

will keep writing down my thoughts and

The progress continues to occur.

Yes, today is Saturday and the date is 25

August 2012.

What has happened since I last wrote?

I'll try to be detailed and explain

as much as I can so you understand my

State of mind during this time.

My days usually start at 05.30-06.00

then they should cancel itself out of bed with the help of

the left arm and left leg.

During the morning hours is right

Page more or less unusable.

When I came up in a sitting position is

It's time to try to get up out of bed and get

the balance of the body to be able to

move to the wheelchair.

Once you have the balance
starts fine

balance between bed and
wheelchair with

small tentative steps and I
need to know after

Very carefully before I move
on the right leg.

This procedure must be
completed every morning so

It is routine.

I have to also look at your
right foot before I

moving the leg.

This is because feelings on the
heels and toes of

right foot doesn't work and as
we all know

control your toes the balance
of bone so this is a

very important moment.

When I finally have dragged
myself to

the wheelchair starts a last
trip to the bathroom

with toilet visits and more a difficult

task of the shower.

Shower is a pretty tricky task with one

Functioning arm and one good leg.

Equipment that is a must in a custom

bathrooms are as follows.

A requirement is handle by the toilet and in the

The shower and a shower stool as well.

Well, toilet bowl usually act as

undressing site before the
shower because it is

only place that is low enough,
so you

can reach all the way to the
floor to

remove both socks, pants and

Underwear.

To get from the toilet bowl to
the shower should

I use the crutch if it is
unsteady,

but I tend to move me but.

Thus the left foot forward,
then easily lug

Right foot, slowly but surely
into the shower corner

And drag for shower curtain.

Washing and further details be omitted

Because it is individual for each person.

To find their own way to succeed in this

feat.

When we finished we
showered and dried out

reasonably dry, it's time to try

Start dressing themselves and this

Item takes about an hour.

Sitting in a wheelchair, we must begin by

try to get in the right arm in
the right sleeve of the
sweater

"which is not easy" because
the arm is completely useless

and without sensation.

 When successful, push in

the head of the shirt and
finally stops the

the left arm.

When this is done it starts a bit hard

Bit to get the shirt over the shoulder and back.

This subsection does not sound so complicated but bear in

given that you've just showered and the body is easy

moist.

Add to you no feeling on the right side so

Therefore, any operation should be done with the left arm.

Try ourselves sometime so I can give you the feeling of

How bloody awkward it can be.

Well then follows the fun element with

underwear and pants.

The principle is similar but we must lift and

Drag a bit at a time, but in the end it was also

fitted underwear and pants.

Pooh!

Hard is it: but now there only

socks and shoes and the mounts to the

as follows, while the sock in
his left hand and

open it with thumb and
forefinger wood the

Over the foot. First the right
and then the left.

That a boy, now remains only
the shoes to be dressed

for the day's activities.

When it comes to my shoes so
I have been learning

me one hand tighing.

This means that you get wood
if shoe lace then

To make a fast knot in one
end of the string.

End with attached wooden in
the upper

the left side of the shoe and
then you take the string
around the

the road to the last hole on
the right side and follow the

then just holes cross-as usual the whole

the way up.

You can now begin to assemble the shoe on the foot.

 the right foot and to me that means a shoe and a

plastic strip down for the foot's ability to control matters.

One can easily get in the foot and I pull for quite

hard for stability.

To be able to tie a knot with one

hand pulling to as usual but at top

overlap, stop a small loop in the

and then for you through another loop

Through the first and tighten.

Now I tied my shoes and is ready to

go out and meet the staff for today's first coffee.

After coffee and breakfast,
which I also Cook

self-rolling, I now turn to the
elevator too go

The top two floors to the
training room.

Yes, exercise.

Well then I'll tell you what I do for that

bring back my body functions in full,

Or those good things are going to get them.

I always start my training with the wheelchair

in front of a wide table in front of me.

This is to be able to carry out this morning's first task.

I begin by setting up the damaged

the arm on the table with a crocheted pot holder during the hand.

Then I grabbed the right wrist and pulls out right arm fully.

First straight ahead to the left and right

side of the table and stretching out my arm as much as possible.

This step is repeated about ten times.

Then it's time for the wrist and hand with fingers.

Using the left hand tie each

I straighten out fingers to maintain

The tenderness in all joints.

 After this pass, so it's time for

nerve stimulation which occurs with a ball of

rubber, which has long tags and

This wonderful ball does wonders.

One wheel simply over arm shoulder, hand.

First at the top then the bottom for best effect.

Massage with the ball about 15minuter.

Now it's time for a little harder but

very important arm workout.

It performs I by two cuffs

With a piece of string between them.

String running across a small wheel and is in my case

Attached at the top of a rib frame.

This training equipment is available with both silent

and elastic line, in my required a silent line of

best muscle workout.

The elastic rope becomes way too wobbly and

the risk of injury increases
significantly because no

concrete movement is
obtained.

I range one cuff on right

arm and rolls into the
wheelchair with back first

to rib frame and grab then the other

The cuff with the left hand.

Then just drag right arm slowly

but surely against the ceiling and the pressure really out

the arm in full and then release it back

Slowly again and repeat 20 times.

After this arm therapy remain two

moment of my training.

The first is standard stair workouts, which

means go up a flight of stairs and down again

And charged to the right leg as much as possible.

The final part of my daily

training involves regular honest walk in a

Long hallway, four passes roundtrip.

This training I told you now, I run

twice a day, seven days a week.

OK, a little more information about me as a person

is well aware that I'm going through the process with a

mother diagnosed with terminal cancer and

This also affects my consciousness, but this

make me stronger and make me fight even harder.

Then can I mention that even the housing question

up for grabs right now and need to be resolved before last August.

So some stuff also happens around that

affect me mentally and physically, but I

do not allow myself to feel pain or

grief, because they are destructive forces and that

I can't afford.

To conclude with writing this

time, I can say that my time has been

better and Lo and behold, but yesterday the 24

August started two fingers on my right hand

being able to move!

Sure it's not much but they move!

The arm is not dead after all, you can understand how

great this is?

This is what I can tell you today and I

will be back with more news when some time passed.

Today is 27/8.

Has been in the hospital most of the day for

an evaluation and first day at

day rehabilitation.

Evaluation means that they look to the

improvements you had time to do and what you

still having problems with.

In my case is the situation like this:

My arm has no function in above or below

arm, the positive aspect of
the arm is to feel

In the skin come back a little
bit.

Not a feather-light touch, but
with slight pressure

I feel throughout the length and

Your fingers can now move in the hugging motion.

All fingers except the thumb who persist in to play dead.

The current balance is very good and without any fall trends.

Tested like this: Stand feet together and stand completely upright.

Then, close your eyes and you'll try

maintain balance even with your eyes closed

which is not easy.

For me, I can keep the balance for about ten

seconds before I get wobbly and get cases

trends due to stroke.

After this step, it is high time that

check the strength of the body after intense

training for 14 days.

First up is to see how my time has changed

from the beginning it was my time a little bit trailing

And the body leaned very right.

But the results after my training is a non

trailing gait, and far less inclination

Of the body during the walk.

Therefore, summary time and strength

Training has given good results.

In addition to the actual strength part of

Leg, arm and chest muscles.

We start with the bone: my
leg, straightened out

as good as the left with some

Effort, the physiotherapist
was received with slight
pressure.

According to her are leg much
stronger than

in the past, and she has some trouble pressing

received when I press the leg up.

The next step is to squeeze your leg back so

much as you can, the physiotherapist retrying

keep and this particular moment is very exhausting for me.

This is because the muscles that will be

push backwards does not work quite as they should,

so the power is much lower but however

Stronger than for 14 days ago.

Foot on the right side has
from the beginning been a

problems, and not much
change has taken place

there.

I have the strength to push
forward, but some muscles

lack the power to pull the foot
up against

the body.

So summary is: movement ability in

the leg has improved a great deal which is

very positive.

Movement of the foot is, unfortunately, in large

Unchanged which is not a good sign.

Now I ordered to go and put me on

 back at the brits in the gymnastics Hall, they want to look

a little more on body balance.

Thus lying on your back, pull
up both legs

To the bent knee position and
both feet down at bench.

Assemble the legs and bend
both legs first to

right and then to the left side,
do this

item two times.

Then, lift your pelvis/buttocks
from bunk

with leg help twice, at this

moment I am weaker on the
right side, so the cod-end

Get a little unsteady initially.

But I manage nonetheless perform two lift.

Now to the final examination of my

Evaluation and for my right foot.

I will be asked to remove the
shoe and foot frame

from the leg as I do, the test
starts with

the staff's help, I will now
push the foot

Down as much as I can.

Which leads to a downward movement with about five

centimeters.

Now, I am told to pull the foot up, which

Do not give any movement at all.

This is because the muscles that

controls the tilt ability are not
Working at all.

She now wants me to touch
the toes on my

Right foot which does not
lead to anything at all.

Summary is that the foot is and probably

remains partially paralyzed because there is no sense of touch

see either the heel or toes, and there is also

No power to perform the tilt feature.

Another test sequence was carried out concerning

the stubborn right arm and went like this:

The first step is to add an unknown subject

in the right hand Palm and you

close my eyes throughout the test, with the help of

the left hand should you now identify the object.

Known throughout the hand and can

way to produce if the subject is cold or warm

the form in which it has
roughly and on surface

is hard or soft, this is no easy
task

because I have almost no
sensation at all inside

the hand.

Further in the arm test is so I
try to straighten out

my arm with only muscle
power, which becomes

a big fiasco because no force,
see

neither over or forearm.

Summary is that the hand can move four

fingers "very good" over and under arm

have no power "more training required" axis

and shoulder have power and are strong which is

very good.

This is the assessment that is the basis

for further referral to the regional hospital in Orebro.

Now over to day rehabilitation and the

includes largely just to hang out with you people.

 others in the same situation and coffee and a little more

training.

Well today, it is the 23rd September 2012.

Yes, it's been a while since I wrote something as a

Some changes have taken place to date.

Then out from short time accommodation in

Degerfors, I have now lived with my brother in

A few weeks ' time.

What has changed?

Since I wrote the last movement in both hand

and arm improved significantly, the hand can now touch all five fingers.

Movement is limited unfortunately of aches and

Swelling in both hand and wrist.

The wrist can bend up and
down max 5

times since the exhaustion
and cannot more.

Hand's fingers are capable
know of to squeeze

easy stuff around but not with
force enough to

clip or lift, the biggest concern is

However, letting go, then, straighten the fingers.

On physical gymnastics, we have continued training

with both arm and leg along with

balance.

The training we do with arm is that I

lying on your back to lift the
arm from lying

to resting on the elbow, but
that neither

Wobble or fall back. "Trust me
this is

not an easy task!

When I finally, with the help
of the eyes

stabilized his arm in this
position, will now

the next challenge to from
elbow mode press

arm up towards the ceiling
and this my friends

Manage maybe once out of 10 attempts.

We see this as a very simple thing but

After a stroke, it is a very difficult

task, we know his arm and
shouting at the in

its interior to rise up against
the ceiling as it usually
ignores.

This is and feels very
frustrating but

is a very important part of the
exercise to regain

Control of your nerves and muscles again.

If we manage to reach toward the ceiling, it is

 an achievement unparalleled to give absolutely everything

in order to do this.

Then follow further exercises, with the arm in

Arm bow mode I'll now try to tilt it

backward against the staff's
hand and touch at

and then back to the original
position

again, it goes with the
tenacity and strength but it

Eating away at the forces.

After this step remains a
further and

It is from the elbow position
let the arm

slowly sit down to the
stomach without falling

And then back to the original position again.

These exercises will be repeated as many times as

you drop, then if you drop out these

exercises at home which also improve on your own

mobility.

OK on to the leg.

Since I wrote last, some happened even at

This area my sensation has improved in both

leg and foot.

The leg has obviously become more powerful and capable

by both stairs and longer walks without

major problems with the help of crutch when walking further.

of course, but the balance has become a little better and

Therefore, my time.

The continued training of the leg consists of

walking and standing on a balance cushion, a

balance cushion is a rubber cushion intended for

both feet filled with some sort
of jelly for

to be varied.

Standing on this balance
cushion do I now

try to stand completely still,
which is not easy with

given the reduced sensation
and balance

on the right side, but we have run this exercise

a few times now and I think at present to

It runs really good.

Another exercise on this pillow is to

Standing on this, I will now
close your eyes and

maintain balance and this is a
very

difficult moment because my
balance is much decreased

with eyes that do.

I close my eyes and try to
balance the

runs fine at first, then I know
of cases

the tendency to the right time
I stood on the pillow

 corresponds to ten seconds
and that's what I

pass now.

So as you probably already understand, this is a

I am very unhappy with the results but it

is unfortunately in the condition my balance is in

the State of play.

This exercise is part of a test that is to

basis for further referral to the central hospital in Orebro.

Another exercise includes the following:

Seated in a regular Chair without arm rests will

I drive myself without using
the fresh

arm and go a short trip turn
and go

back to the Chair and put me
softly without using

the hand.

This is done on time and my time was last

34 seconds and is quite good considering

I go slowly and have poor balance not

true?

Oh well on to the next care namely

 the foot.

It has been a major concern since the start

But even here, the improvements brought to the

position, previously I had no sensation in either

toes or heel.

This has been improved in the sense that I have

started feeling in right big toe and the foot's wiggle

function has been greatly improved and I can

Now bend the foot both upwards and downwards.

Bending the foot upwards are still not without

trouble and can't bend fully, but it can

at least give in both up and down

This is a great achievement!

Nursing gymnastics is now tailored to me

improvements and emphasis is put on the balance

and walking exercise.

I am also asked to cycle on
exercise

cycle on physical gymnastics
in order to maintain

both breathing and fitness of
the body and when

I bikes I usually use some sort of

glove for right hand, because it does not

Can grab and hold the handlebars by itself.

This glove looks like a long

leather glove with Velcro fastener on wrist

and in the front is what a long tongue, when

put your hand on the handle bars is this

heavy and pulls over your hand and thus becomes

hand completely encased in a glove and you

stuck at the handlebars.

Pretty clever, in fact, if I may say so

itself.

Well so far so good now to
the

refractory foot that always
has a tendency to

will rotate to the right, this is
solved by using

by an elastic band that strains
over your foot

And attached to the pedal of bike.

OK now we're ready to pedal away about ten

minutes by 1.5 Joule's load tends to be

fully sufficient training then you have trampled about

three kilometers.

Then as each day's training, I usually step

out of the wheelchair and have it in front of me to support

for a hearty walk both on the flat straight road

But even in crates to get resistance.

In the evenings I usually go up and down in

the stairs of my brother with the help of

the handrail usually tries to go up and down

the stairs three times and the stairs is made up of 16

steps.

I also have all the training schemes

health care written out to me and used

On a daily basis to achieve maximum results.

Tomorrow Monday, it's another day on the

day rehabilitation that awaits with more

training, on Tuesday following a doctor's visit on

regional hospital in Orebro for my final

evaluation and then emerges from me

The ability to drive a car again and so on.

Time for my doctor's visit was postponed to

on September 29 on Friday because of

double booking for patients.

Yes, my friends today say the calendar to

the date is September 30, 2012 and I

 have completed my visit at the doctor at

regional hospital in Orebro.

What emerged?

The doctor did a thorough inspection of me

opportunities to be able to move my leg, arm, foot

with the following results.

My leg can move relatively well both forward

and backwards but have distinct spasms at

load but also difficult to maintain balance

By motion to the side.

This does, of course, my time and

the doctor does not believe this will change

significantly in the future.

My arm has been improved in terms of strength to

lift and hold it up for a long
while, no

much difference with regard
to squeeze and release

The grip on a mug or a pen.

When you try to grab a mug I
get strong

pain in the wrist and this
makes it impossible

to try to keep and draw my
hand than.

 less to grab the mug, this
depends on the

weakening in both wrist and
to the muscles

has thinned out considerably.

According to the doctor, this
will be coached

up to a certain degree but will probably

Never be really good again.

My right foot Yes, it has been a

concern for himself and now it can be said that the

works fine after the
conditions I have

for it, the foot is able to bend
both up and

down to constrained modes,
turning the foot in

Lateral work to the left but
not to the right.

Contributing to the foot
would like to turn to the

right in the time ahead, so my
goal should be to

try to keep your foot straight
at the time and not over

strain at normal walk.

Regarding the sensation in the foot is missing it in right

page on the above page, and almost all of the

The underside of the foot.

These mobility problems that remain can be difficult

If not impossible to work out, but I get

Learn to live with them during the time the

the body tries to heal which is a

process that can take years to achieve.

Additional information resulting from

doctor's visit was that my
facial paralysis

not lost but are still present
and causes

Some speech problems, and
according to the doctor reads

This clinical picture aphasia
which is

speech impairment.

Then it emerged that my eyes do not

keep up with reaction in following

a finger as the doctor holds up in front of you

and move sideways and up
and down, my eyes

React but not fast enough.

So with these factors added to my

current situation does not directly cause

easier to deal with but I have no

Choice but to keep fighting.

Within 14 days, I get further information from

Orebro if I will be inserted on the

Rehabilitation Department or if I won't.

will have to take a taxi between three days per

week, this is the information I have included

and also you readers as I write

down the information I myself is notified.

This and my further fortunes do I tell at

a later time.

For you people out there who doubted me

ability to recover me so sorry I am

stronger than you thought, and for those of you who think

I set high goals, I can only say

I always aim for the stars and I will reach my goals.

Finally, a Word to your others in the same situation: aim for the stars and always continue to fight large

Hugs to you all.

A final thank you to the following wards

with Staff.

Central Hospital in Karlstad emergency room/stroke

Ward

Karlskoga hospital Ward 1A

Västergården in Degerfors.

Nursing gymnastics at Karlskoga hospital

A big thank you to all of you, without you I would not be here.

Where I am today I bow deeply to you all.

Thanks to you readers and who knows maybe we get in touch again.

With a warm greeting.

P. Raven.

Resurgence 2.

The Quest for Freedom.

Author: Peter. T. Raven.

Yes, my good friends today
say the date

Tue 6 November and I was
going to continue

tell you about further
progress since

the month of September.

Since I last wrote, I've continued

with my training in the nursing gymnastics in

Karlskoga two days per week Mon and

Thursdays with effective training time on two

And a half hours per day.

My training has mostly been about

balance and strength-building

both legs and arm also some strength training

For the right foot has been included.

But ok, we go into it a little closer up as we usually do.

Balance training has mostly been about

stand on one leg at a time, first the left and

then the right the left leg is no

problems whatsoever.

The right, on the other hand,
have great difficulty

to be able to carry the entire

body weight of itself it is
capable of

Its height just over five to ten
seconds during load.

On balance exercises have taken place with a

balance disc and it consists of a round

disc in either wood or plastic with grooved

pattern so it will not slip, centered in

the center of its underside a

Ridge that makes when it is in plant

so are you free from the floor by using the

your own balance.

This is an art piece in itself and with

reduced sensation in both legs and feet make it

all the easier, my biggest problem, however, is

I miss feel completely in the heel of the right

Feet and has only little sensation in the foot's toes.

This affects the outcome, of course, but

I can proudly say that I know

can both stand steadily without falling for

page and can handle even making knee

Bends without losing my balance.

The problem with trying to
get the plate to

Lean first then backward and
from side

to the side is, of course, the
absence of sensation in the

toes and heels I know simply
was not

the foot is and how it is positioned to one hundred

percent.

A further task is the result when

the case of standing balance and its game Console Wii.

With the help of the game and applications

is to keep balance as

for example, go on line is very difficult

Since you are using your own body

to balance the figure's slant on the wire

without falling down, yet another challenge

available in the game when you're almost half

Road nothing against you

and you are going to simulate a jump both feet together

To avoid to fall from the rope.

I can say that this game is not easy to

do even for people with full function but for

us with reduced, it is almost impossible

Although obviously it's a great workout.

No. I did not manage to complete the game.

Well in balance we have also

tried to train up the creek and

Cross back balance and it goes to like this.

Lying on my back on a wide bunk with the head on a pillow now staff hand me

a large rubber ball like thing

though this is a little different it is more

elongated and a section on the middle looks

as they tightened the belt hard at a

large rubber ball.

Well it looks like and lying on your back

adding up both legs on

increases and should then with leg

help lift both buttocks and
lumbar so

High as it will go.

This exercise should be
repeated five times

You can keep up.

When it comes to myself so I
can not

lift the right and left sides as high due to

to the right side is weaker after stroke

but I can nevertheless, lifting her ass from

bunk five times and that's what

The exercise is all about.

An item remains in the
subject balance

training and standing without

fall with the left foot placed
on a round

Plastic ball and this sounds
easy isn't it?

Remember that this is not the
case now remember that

the right leg is difficult to clear the whole

the body's weight and then have the fresh

foot on a subject who would like to roll away.

This is an almost impossible task

the record for myself is only five seconds.

Yes, that's what we train in the balance

In addition to normal walking without a crutch of course

and to go after a line on the floor a foot

After the other on the same route, the same

principle to go on line but with a

line painted on the floor instead.

It was balance it.

Strength training then.

We start well with the bone because it is

What makes the best progress?

The training has mainly consisted in

machine training in addition to balance parts

and have been following.

We have trained leg kick which means you

sitting in a machine that has two well stuffed

pillows in front of each leg and there is a

Substantial weight stacks to choose from.

Your task now is to press your legs outwards

to the fully extended position
and then slowly

back with as much weight as
possible and

with both leg help did I just
over

Eighty kilograms in ten
repetitions.

But to make matters more difficult

I was told to use only the right

leg and we started with 10 kg in five

iterations, this went well we are raised to

15 kg and drove five repetitions it

still went well.

I told the staff to increase to twenty

5 kg which they did and it went well

It was getting a bit vibrato with the return

That should be done slowly and constricting.

We raised to 30 kg and I passed the five

duplication here but now it started

receive on both the front and back movement

and your right knee will be spasticity at this load.

Oh sorry for those of you who don't know what spastic

means it is when the leg will slow up a movement peacefully but the leg

Instead, the brake releases

repeatedly with no control

that is what is meant by spastic movement.

After this spastic movement patterns

I felt now that I wanted to test how much

weight my right leg actually managed so

we loaded on 40 kg and I passed

Still the importance of certain problems and five repetitions.

This pleased me greatly and we loaded now

fifty kilograms as resistance I
sat down

grips swaged and as much as I
could

inducing but this heaviness
was simply too

much at least for now.

The next leg is similar

exercise but here you should
press

the legs forward then leg
presses as much

you cope with varying weights

Resistance.

This machine I have tried
before, so

I know that with both leg
force capable

I whole registry with weights,
which means

one hundred forty kg in total,
but this is irrelevant.

What would be tested now it was right

leg strength and motion control, so we

started with 20 kg for ten repetitions and

It went without complaint.

We thus continued with 30 kg and

nor was that any problem we increased

further to 40 kg and now it started

become a hassle for my right knee that wanted that

usually pump braking on the way back

Which may not take place?

We decided to increase further to 50 kg

and it got really heavy for my right leg

but I pushed myself too clear the

10 the rehearsal that was the goal to

The weight would be approved.

But ok 50 kg is what my leg is capable of

In leg press right now.

On the strength training have I tried to

train my right foot by first working out

with weights and I am ashamed almost to tell that right foot only passes a Resistance on a kg is not a little bit more.

So instead of weights, we have tried two

more methods one includes a

rubber string to draw around
your foot in

Height with upper foot pad.

Then, hold against yourself
while you

try to press your feet down
and this is

much harder than it sounds,
and just

This exercise was not
particularly effective

for my part, because my right
foot well

would writhe on the left
under load,

and this led simply to

The rubber band slipped off
my foot.

So a new way to work out the
foot was a

need of physiotherapists had

found an old tool that would

Help me in this work.

The gear is a very simple

construction with two foot plates with

non-slip, of course, and during "the pedals

"two pretty heavy duty coil springs and in

the bottom one wooden plate to stand firmly on the

the floor.

Therefore, a simple design that would

Prove to be a real success.

My task is to put both feet on the

pedals and simply press down and hold back on the way back, very simple and very effective I used to train with this tool from fifteen minutes up to 30 minutes.

This tool, I recommend hot

To all of you who train out there.

OK wow what I nag haha.

But actually I think it's fun to

write and I share more than happy with me

of the experiences I had and what

I itself has benefited greatly from

Hope you don't mind.

Well what can I tell you more right now?

Well it clearly arms and hand should we not

forget, of course, we have been training them

with.

To begin with, I would like to tell you about what

progress made and how we maintain

Mobility and softness in all joints.

Firstly, my hand and arm

become stronger muscle wise and it has

contributed to more mobility for both arm and

care.

In order to maintain
smoothness and mobility in

my fingers as I sit and bending

soft in a hugging motion and

then slowly, carefully
straighten them completely

I do this on a daily basis
mainly morning and

evening but even on days when I have

While over.

This is good for both to maintain

movement and softness of your finger

results should also be massaging both fingers

and hand and movement but also for

sense of touch.

Arm and shoulder also need them

relaxation this is done by

lift both shoulders toward the ceiling and relaxes

of repeat ten times, the arm relaxed

by sitting with a table in front of

themselves.

Stretch out your arm in its entire length first straight

out and then to the right and left

page in smooth movements repeat ten times

Once this is done, leave the arm of own

power move up toward your mouth and slowly

Back down repeat ten times.

OK now we're soft and heated nice

isn't it?

So what has improved since last time?

In my arm, it has not so much been

more than that, it has become a bit more sensitive to

touch and that it gathered
more strength and

can withstand more exercises
without

Slowing as fast as before.

My shoulder still teasing
taunts on

me with hurt and leading
ports a little out

the led on the night which
leads to poor sleep

and of course, pain.

The solution to this concern
believe

physical therapists that it is
mantilla which is

a blue fabric similar band with Velcro

fastening set with one end is made to a

loop and place it over the right arm buttoning

To lie down at the elbow.

Then the rest of the mantilla be

Over your back against the left shoulder and over the

another loop is done in this end with

Velcro mount if you rated it over

left shoulder you will now put your right hand in

the loop you created in this way have your now

arranged a relief for right shoulder and arm.

I'm told to use the mantilla.

daily and try to follow these

instructions but sometimes makes it quite

simply to painful to be able to wear it, but

as I have said, listen always on staff they

Usually know what is needed.

Over to my right hand.

Changes that have taken place there is the following.

I can now bend the four out
of five fingers

little finger on the hand did
not want to work

Since day one, it is not much
to say

The more gratifying is that the
thumb index and

middle finger can both bend
over and even

straighten out its own power
which was not

the case in September in
which they could bend

But not straight at all.

Progress thus Similarly, now me

wrist got better than it was in

September it can now bend over both

up and down, but due to the continued

swelling is load still a

Problem.

Some might have been added in his hand but

not enough to pin and

Keep solid object while I go.

What has been more?

Well I had set up a personal goal to

able to go one kilometer with a crutch and it

I hit by far not so long ago

then I decided that being that take a

walk of just over three and a half

kilometers.

So this limit I have beaten by a wide margin would

I probably say.

Without the crutch I would think that I can handle

Probably five hundred meters at present.

Indoors I go without a crutch at all times

But outdoors, it is a must.

As I told you in the previous book so

We carried out a lot of tests regarding

speed from sitting to

turn around, etc.

These tests were done as recently as the first

November 2012 again and I have improved

the results of all tests and this makes

me incredibly happy because it is something

There is no notice under

Training periods.

First November 2012 was also my last

today on sick gymnastics in Karlskoga and

I just want to say a big thank you to all of you

you have been wonderful and very helpful non mentioned and non-forgotten.

You know who you are.

My new training camp is now

Orebro University Hospital.

Where did I first day 5 November in

year and what I've seen of it so far

seems to be very promising both staff

and also training opportunities.

My new physical therapist examined me

carefully so we know which muscles and joints as

working and which ones need
extra training but some need
training only

To a greater or lesser degree.

My new occupational
therapist has informed me

me about what is to come in

development of the ability and the

both woodwork and kitchen service

means to learn to Cook, bake make coffee etc.

Therefore, such things as are necessary for

To live at home in a normal environment.

The next minor surprise came of her desire me to return the

wheelchair with the comment it needs you No longer since you walk so well.

I thought to myself do I do that?

But in all honesty, she has a great

part right for my wheelchair is most of the time

still either at home or in the hospital so

It does no direct benefit for me.

So in the morning before I go to Orebro to go in to the gymnastics and return it and only keep the crutch for future support.

This is what can be written right now

but of course I will come back again soon

With more news for you.

Today is November 15, 2012 and

Some have occurred since I last wrote

So we continue will tell.

Since I wrote last, my daily

activities in Karlskoga ceased and

I have moved over to day

rehabilitation in Orebro.

The first thing that happened was that it was

introduced to both staff and with patients and then the usual

Tour.

After introduction, it was time for all

paper with the training schedule and

General information.

My schedule is as follows me

days begin 07.20 then my taxi come to pick

me up for trip to Karlskoga hospital where I

Must wait for service line to Orebro.

For those of you who don't know what Service line

is I can tell you it is a small bus to transport patients between hospitals

Karlskoga and Orebro hospital without fee.

So then a 30-minute wait at

Service line in Karlskoga after the

over to Orebro and the journey takes

approximately 40 minutes to one hour

Depending on how many you want to get

Picked up and what driver it is.

So at nine time or shortly thereafter

I tend to be on the site but my day

do not start until 10.30 o'clock so

There is plenty of time for a coffee break before

the day begins.

This particular gap, I have talked to

the staff and I will probably

Start at 10 in the future.

Well my day begins at present

with a pass physical therapy followed by a

Pass with occupational therapy since lunch

followed by another then

physical therapy and occupational therapy which

End my day at 14.30 hours.

Service line is home to 15:00 and I am

at the hospital in Karlskoga at approximately

16:00 time and my connection taxi

home will not until 16.40 so unfortunately

much of my time goes away in travel time and

At home, I am home at 17 and trust me then you are completely finished.

Oh good back to training and work therapy in Orebro.

Firstly, I would like to mention that I'm not

use the wheelchair further and the decision was made together with the therapy and physiotherapy.

How it goes?

Well actually really good leg becomes

 stronger and stronger day by day and

I'm out and walking about three

kilometers per day whether I'm

Free or not.

So for those of you out there who are struggling and it

seems pointless never stop fighting

each thing you do will help much more than

you believe and you will succeed if you

set small goals all the time I know

I did it myself.

So my only companion on the road

Now is Mr. crutch and we will continue the path together and has worked

Very well so far but.

Unfortunately, it will be
replaced next

week towards a more modern
red with

soft ergonomic handle.

I have also submitted the application for

both the disability allowance and car allowance

and now await only a medical certificate to

Add and precisely it can be

difficult to obtain but shock on the whole

Time to give those with him.

Yes, I have tried to drive a car already

and it runs really good but the one that I

going to buy must get some reconstruction

for the problem with my right hand and arm.

The problems in the right arm and the hand is probably caused by an injury

which I do not remember that I done to me but according to the doctor, it is something broken.

So this Friday November 16

starting my day with an x-ray and a

meeting with the surgeon.

The same day, I have a scheduled

meeting with the hospital's neurons psychologist

who wants to talk to me for two hours so

my morning workout disappears completely

but I've still have my own

Afternoon sessions as luck would have it.

Training sessions consists of the following torque.

First I'm starting my pass with five

minute warm-up on training

cycle with 1, 5 kgp resistance and may

using the staff to bind fixed me

right hand on the handlebars and my right foot at pedal.

This is because the hand is not strong

enough to hold on to the handlebars and foot

turning toward the crankset.

Yes, we continue to the next station and

This is to work out the right arm with

using a device attached to a bench

and weights I'll explain.

It takes place on the bench
and places

right arm in something that
looks like a

long Crescent formed support
for arm

and at the end a grip handle,

the handle is sitting on a position that is

adjustable for best adaptation.

At the front there is a loop that moves weights

can be attached and in my case only one kilo

for the time being.

It takes place on the bench and put

arm in support and grip the handle

but I get the same way tight fast my hand around the handle bar to be able to work out at all.

Staff will help me with it and also

To hook in weight on the handle.

We must now bring his hand
and

the arm that working towards
the body so

many times as possible and it
is

tall order despite the low
weight but

the hardcover and shoulder does still hurt but the exercise must

implemented for training's sake and for

Continued movement of the arm.

The following station is the leg press.

This machine is a construction man

step into and grips and

at the front there is a large foot plate of

aluminum which is attached to a

adjustable weight stacks.

My exercise to gouge both

legs to almost fully extended mode

with a weight resistance on 40 kg and

This is repeated 30 times for my part.

Now over to the bar and sitting

training.

Lying on your back should I now raise both

arms over head as far as it will go without doing pain and it can be a bit tricky given sore arm and shoulder.

But this should be done in my case 2 x 10 times and it is a huge effort but necessary for

The bodies further operation.

Now in a sitting position, I will now take

up your shoulders towards your ears and then

slowly lower them down again and this

Repeat 2 x 10 times.

Further exercises in prone position Is the following.

Laying on back bend both legs and

put them down in the couch when you have bent

knees and from this location you should now

fold one leg to the side while you

hold the other stable in bunk

Repeat 2 x 10 times each leg.

We continue with the pelvic lift.

Lying on your back, you should now

Lift

the tail from bunk and lower slowly

back this operation is repeated 2 x 10

times.

Another exercise while lying on the back.

To now trail the entire leg to the side

your toes should point toward the ceiling all the time

And the leg should not be lifted from the couch.

This step is repeated 3 x 5 times.

The training session ends with a

Seated exercise and it is as follows.

Add up the right leg in its
entire length

on the couch and fall
forwards in

the hip until the strain is felt
in the back

thigh hold about 30 seconds
and

then do the same with the

left leg.

You will see my workouts three days

per week but note that two days

This week is the twin such that.

Sure it's tough and very

frustrating but if you that I own

the stubbornness, it will

very well to use during this

training.

OK moving on to occupational therapy.

Yes, for one, starts working therapy

to sit at a table with a

towel under my arm and working

forward and to the sides about five to

Ten minutes to loosen up your joints.

Since I usually use me by

a soft tag ball to stimulate

The nerves of the hand and arm.

Now we're going to try to do something specific

of it all.

At the time of writing I have not had time

try on so much yet but I have

tried to get up and place

around Styrofoam ball and place them on

A Board with the intended hole.

The most recent result was 20 balls in

various sizes placed and removed

Picked which is a good result.

Then I tried to unscrew the

a plastic nut from a plastic screw

worse results because the hand does not

Capable of turning just squeezing.

I should add that I have big problem

with movement in my hand because of

Swelling and poor blood circulation.

This will be checked up on Friday 16th

November and I hope of course that

It is possible to solve in any way regardless of

If it means surgery.

So my training in the field of occupational therapy is

limited but the balls, I will

continue with because it trains both

grip and release movement of the hand and the

More training, the stronger it becomes.

This pass is run twice daily two

times a week and I have pretty high hopes for myself.

Well this is what I can write just now but I will be back a little later

with more information about what

happening and what is planned ahead

for one, both in terms of training and

occupational therapy and also

insurance I will keep you

Informed I promise.

Friday 16 November. Yes, today has the

been full speed but not quite what I

expected by day.

I found myself at the hospital at about

09.15 and made it with a cup of coffee

then I was told by the nurse

that right after lunch I would at

x-rays of my hand and wrist at

because of the swelling and pain from

hand and wrist.

But first, I have an appointment with the neuron

psychologist between 10 and 12 and his

Job is the following.

He picked up various drawings

I would copy to see how well

the brain is capable of this

the task, then rattled off a

list of words and you'll repeat the

He speaks the words he read 15 words

and I was able to reproduce the five or six

pieces.

This list was read up about five

times and I could remember

about five or six words each

time, then, he read up further

a list of 15 words and the result was

like, in conclusion, he read up

all words with a new involved and

I would render the words I recognized

and say in which of the first two

lists they were or if they were not there

with at all, and which I managed to better

Would think about 15 words properly positioned.

More information was to delete numbers from

a mixture of numbers and to follow

lines between bullets and numbers, and

do I need to add that it was time to

All test.

This was what we had time on our two

hours.

A new meeting with him is scheduled

on Monday next week for further

tests and there will also be a

third meeting focusing on car

Run time.

OK now we take lunch!

The time now is 12:30 pm and
I'm on my way

for emergency Radiology
reception and well

in place so it was my hand
carefully

studied and they quickly saw
that it was

abnormally swollen and
fingers and

wrist hard to bend.

So they x-rayed first hand with

fingers from both above and in

side to side then came wrist from above

and from the side since I was asked

To wait in the waiting room at the result.

The nurse came a bit later and

explained to me that the result had

sent directly to my doctor by computer

And I could go back to the rehabilitation.

So I had to take the crutch and

wander back to the Division where

the nurse met me and told me I

have time for some therapy before

ends for the day.

OK then, only to wander away to

Nursing gymnastics then met me

physical therapist myself and we started

with a bit of arm bends into the machine I

described in the past but I can not

many because of pain in the arm

and shoulder.

Well she thought we skip the arm and

walking on the leg press
instead and I

drove my 30 repetitions on 40 kg

then I said that I wanted to feel on the

the weight of 50 kg and did even 10

repetitions with the weight.

So will continue the weight of

Leg press be 50 kg nothing else.

We went to the bench for exercise

that is to lie on your back with

knees bent and one leg to the side

While the other stays stable.

This is repeated ten times
each leg and

There were no major
problems then became

I asked to put me up on

the edge of the bench with
your feet on the floor.

My physical therapist then mounted a

ten-kg weight on my right leg and asked

me extend it fully and repeat

torque 10 times which I

Managed.

Good, she said, and placed more

a ten-kg weight on my left leg now

We go every two legs starting with the left

running ten then switch to the right and run

Ten repetitions which I did.

She asked if I tried to be

on your toes? I answered no because I

had not tested this item so we

went to the barren and there I had to go up

on your toes 10 times very good, she said it

may suffice for today.

After this hectic day, it became

journey home again at 15 and one hour

While waiting for the connection taxi to

come all the way home so we may ensure

week what is going on, we heard then.

OK here we go since then has the following occurred.

Last Monday the 19/11 got

I granted the hospital journeys by private taxi

because no taxi was booked on me.

morning with the result that I

missed the service line.

On Wednesday it was training in normal

courses with a little extra in the morning

because I start at 10 instead

Ten and thirty.

But then last Thursday came a heavy

notice we were asked to immediately travel

to Uppsala to our mother's cancer

had become much worse, so we did

us ready and went by car there.

I and my siblings sat on the wake of

our mother almost 24 hours a day so

very little sleep there was and our dear

mother fought in the last days to be

here, but on Saturday 24/11 2012 found

She finally peace and she is very

missed by us all.

Rest in peace beloved mom.

I will of course continue me

training and my struggle to get

back but this event will

of course, to reflect in me

continuing struggle.

My priority right now is to find a

home ownership because in
these times

pass neither I nor my siblings
to

be around each other we all
need peace

and quiet and that is why it is
a must to

arrange your own accommodation at any time during the

next week.

So dear readers I will return later

with more information about what

happening around me and of course I'll

mention when this was written today is the

Sunday 25/11 2012.

Yes, today is 27/11 2012 and it

has not been so much more about

training I have done 6 minutes

walking test which means you go in a

corridor which is 25 meters long back and

back as many times as you want on

six minutes.

My case I managed to go six
rounds, then,

300 meters around then I had
to

stop because I was tired and

balance bad and my right foot

drops and get stuck in the
floor which

Risk stumbling and falling.

After the test, we agreed that

My foot contraption do I use
the full

time and I need to practice
my thighs

muscles a lot we tried even to

get up on your toes which
goes with great

difficulty.

As you probably understand,
it is difficult

to find your desire in the
present

circumstances so I will for this

Time to tell a little joyful news.

My efforts to get the drive again

seems to be coming true body

wise, I have the strength and the application is

submitted to the social insurance office if

car allowance and the only document I

need is the physician's assessment and

the I will require tomorrow then

I just need to wait for the decision of the

the social Insurance Agency.

So, with these words I end this

Part 2 of the return but a final part Will OF Course commence as soon as possible because the series will

Follow me for a year.

I wish you all a very Merry Christmas

And a happy new year 2013.

Of course, a huge thank you for caring

staff and wards in the relevant parts.

I hope we can hear about it in my third and final writing on the return from a stroke big hug to all of you out there and you remember never stop fighting and good luck.

See you in 2013.

With a warm greeting

P. Raven.

Resurgence 3
Looking back.

Author: Peter T Raven.

Hello there again it is a long while since I wrote anything regarding my stroke and recovery from it.

But today that is about to change the year is now 2016 and four years has passed since stroke moment.

In this book I will try to explain my efforts and struggles up to now and try to explain why I think like I do and why it feels like it does.

Well my feeling after stroke is that something is missing inside I am not who I was before the stroke.

I feel present but not really here it sounds strange I know but I feel like an empty Wessel drifting, I don't feel emotion in the same way as before.

As I said I am not the person I used to be this edition is brand new to me as well so please be patient.

Me and my family have broken up and I walk alone I can understand why I am not easy to handle my emotions is all over the place.

After stroke I have a hard time showing and receiving emotions of any kind such as love, happiness, sadness, and so on.

Why this is I sadly can't explain I only know that's how things are.

Why I think like I do is also a bit tricky to answer but I will at least try to explain.

Like many other stroke victims, I feel ugly I am good for nothing and I had the urge to end my life what's the point of such existence?

You should all know these thoughts I deal with on a daily basis and this together with constant pain when body does its repairs is not an easy thing to deal with.

But my salvation after stroke is I was granted the talent of writing this is why I continue to write my books it is my way to recover.

Well during the time since I last wrote on the subject many things have happened of course and I will try to tell you as much of it as I can remember.

My body has become much stronger and my brain seem to function fairly well enough to write and do what's expected from me.

I live in my own apartment on the third floor no

elevator so each day is good training in the stair case.

And when it's time for laundry I need to take the clothes down three stairs and outside to neighbor complex where laundry room is fitted.

So laundry is a struggle each time and I am often totally exhausted when it's done.

So I try to do this task once or twice per month since it is rather hard to complete.

The same thing goes for shopping groceries it is very heavy to carry the groceries up three stairs to often.

But I handle everything in my apartment by myself cleaning dishes well everything in the normal household the only issue is that it takes me longer time to complete.

And as many other stroke victims I tend to keep to myself maybe not on purpose I just don't feel like being social sure I can talk to people and hang out at times but it's becoming more and more rare.

For those of you that have read my first two book on the subject stroke know I lost both my parents due to cancer, and in December last year 2015 my biological father died from weak heart.

So during many years I have lost all my older generation and this of course have affected my own rehabilitation.

What remains from my biological family is two brothers and a sister we are the older generation now.

But I know my parents are watching over us all.

Alright enough about this how have I progressed then?

Well as I said my body has become stronger and I can walk without any crutches or other helping supplements and I still drive my own car without issues.

Remember from start I was bed bound with total right side paralysis and went forward to wheel chair and finally stood on my own two legs again freedom at last.

This process has taken the body four years to complete and my doctors are stunned from start he didn't think I ever would walk again, so you can imagine how good it feels to prove him wrong time after time.

Sure I still have some issues such as when out walking I can't walk too fast and my balance makes me to straggle sideways and my right foot still have the tendency to not lift high enough from the street also called drop foot.

My balance also stops me from exercising on in lines and biking which was my passion before stroke occurred.

And another issue is at night when trying to sleep I can wake up from not breathing properly and this have been with me ever since the stroke occurred sounds scary right?

Well yes, it is but after four years I am rather used to it by now and I do have nitro spray in case of inside failures, the only medication I use is anti-blood clothing that's it.

And my condition states that I surely don't need alcohol to be woozy I am each day anyway haha.

During the last six months I deal with an extreme headache which I can't explain but I have a doctor's appointment this month which is September so hopefully they can provide me with further answers to that issue.

For my right arm it can move and grip fairly well but it has little strength still but are improving all the time but will it ever be as before? That is impossible to speculate in just as the right leg and foot.

But looking at the progress the last four years I must say I am pretty proud for what I have accomplished this far.

But as common knowledge says from stroke moment your body has a ten-year time spam to do as much repairs to the damaged areas in the body as possible.

And for me it has past only four and a half years this far so I will continue the fight to regain my mobility maybe not in full but to as good as is possible.

I try to wake up happy each morning but then again what is happy?

I don't plan anything ahead anymore since I am aware that my time on this rock is limited so I take everything on a day to day basis.

Don't get me wrong I am very grateful to still be alive even if it feels no to be fully alive I have four years extra after the stroke that would have killed me if I didn't get the help when I did.

But for how long further I just can't speculate in and I have no desire to find out I will be here for as long as I am allowed to be here that's all.

My goal with my life as it is I want to reach out to the masses and explain a bit about how one can experience the time after a severe stroke attack.

My aim is maybe to be a helping hand to other stroke victims if my books can be an inspiration to others I would be very proud and it would be my honor to help in this manner.

I have been asked to keep seminars at schools and hospitals to talk about stroke and issues related to it but as for now I have declined due to my own rehabilitation.

But I don't say I won't do it ever since I know many people want this information especially from a person with own experience.

But you need to know it is not an easy task to accomplish meeting several hundred people all eager to know all about the event and how you feel and so on but I will try my best to reach that point to help.

Trust me I know there are many stroke victims in the world young and old and the first feeling most of us encounter is we want to quit we don't have the strength to carry on.

To all victims I want to say never ever quit!

Set small goals all the time and always aim at the stars.

Let me give my examples.

From start I was bed bound and I couldn't speak to well due to fascial paralysis my first goal was to be able to communicate so the writing started and at the same time I tried to speak the words I was writing yes it was hard and often the words didn't come out the way it was supposed to but I kept going anyway.

And from the bed I thought I need to fight it's not my

turn to go yet I am not finished.

So in a matter of a week I was presented to my friend the wheel chair and to get up from bed to the wheel chair was a huge step for me.

And with the help from hospital staff I learned to dress myself with only using my left hand and left leg.

Trust my word this is no easy task to accomplish but we humans are remarkable adaptive and we do things as first appear to be impossible.

I was in my wheel chair for almost a year and was in training the whole time and my doctor told me I should not count on walking again due to the gravity of my nerve damages.

His words made me sad and very angry and I told him that we will see I will walk again and I will drive my car again.

He answered me that I should realize how badly injured I was.

His words still ring in my head and they cut deep wounds on my inside and I was ready to give up.

But then my warrior woke up and I thought never I will never quit I will walk again there is no other option so I kept on fighting forcing my body to do almost impossible things.

In the hospital corridors I was training several hours every day in my wheel chair moving forward kicking left leg on the floor and using left arm to gain more speed.

After much training I moved one step closer to walking I was introduced to Mr. Cain so I could stand on my own and try to take some steps not many in the beginning but it increased all the time.

And I had a big smile on my lips inside my head I will show that doctor I thought.

I kept on fighting only to prove him wrong once and

for all I am very stubborn and I pressed my body to its limit every training session.

After about three months I walked fairly well with support from either wheel chair or Mr. Cain.

The doctor was stunned he didn't believe his eyes and I told him never tell me I can't do things because I am too stubborn and I never quit ever.

My training commenced up to the point where I became time to do all the tests to regain my driver's license again I passed all the tests and I did do a driving test with an authorized traffic school teacher and I also passed that test.

I got my license back with two restrictions I must drive an automatic geared car and I must use a steering knob that's all.

So here I was I had sat up my goal one at the time and I aimed to the stars to reach them and guess what? I did reach my goals and if I can I am sure you all can to.

Remember never ever give up always keep fighting even if it seems impossible nothing is impossible we all can adept and always aim at the stars you are stronger than you think.

Sure listen to your doctor but that doesn't mean you have to agree with his words right?

Listen to your own body and your own mind don't let anyone put you down you are stronger than what they think you are use your stubbornness and your inside anger prove them all wrong I know it is very possible.

I know it sounds so easy but
trust me I know the way is
very long and very hard
also painful but you are
actually fighting for you are
you not worth the effort?

Yes, you are always and
forever don't you ever dare
to forget that!

Never ever let the warrior
die you need its strength
and you always need goals
to follow.

My own life today is rather close too normal I manage myself in my own apartment I drive my own car again I have regained my freedom and you can to.

Well for now this is what I can share with you but in time I will return with another book in the subject my best wishes for you all regards Peter. ☺

www.ingramcontent.com/pod-product-compliance
Lightning Source LLC
Chambersburg PA
CBHW070219190526
45169CB00001B/21